OPTIMIZE YOUR GUT HEALTH

A Comprehensive Guide to Healing Leaky Gut with the Ultimate Diet Plan

Adams .U. Morris

TABLE OF CONTENTS

CHAPTER 1

leaky gut diet for food

Leaky Gut Syndrome, often referred to as increased intestinal permeability in medical terms, is a condition that has gained significant attention in recent years due to its potential impact on overall health. In this chapter, we'll dive deep into what exactly Leaky Gut Syndrome is, its causes, the symptoms it can manifest, and why it's crucial to address this condition for your well-being.

Imagine your digestive system as a sophisticated barrier - a wall that separates your bloodstream from the contents of your gastrointestinal tract. This wall plays a vital role in allowing nutrients to enter your bloodstream while blocking harmful substances from passing through. In a healthy gut, this barrier is tight, like a well-constructed brick wall.

However, in cases of Leaky Gut Syndrome, this barrier becomes compromised. It's as if the mortar between the bricks has eroded, allowing unwanted substances to leak through. These substances can include undigested food particles, toxins, and even bacteria. This leakage can have far-reaching consequences for your health.

Causes of Leaky Gut Syndrome

Understanding what causes Leaky Gut Syndrome is essential to addressing it effectively. Several factors can contribute to the development of this condition.

1. **Dietary Choices:** A diet high in processed foods, sugar, and unhealthy fats

can promote inflammation in the gut. This chronic inflammation can weaken the intestinal barrier over time.

2. **Medications:** Some medications, such as nonsteroidal anti-inflammatory drugs (NSAIDs) and antibiotics, can disrupt the balance of bacteria in the gut, potentially leading to Leaky Gut Syndrome.

3. **Chronic Stress:** Prolonged periods of stress can affect gut health. Stress activates the body's "fight or flight"

response, which can influence the permeability of the intestinal barrier.

4. **Infections:** Infections like small intestinal bacterial overgrowth (SIBO) and candida overgrowth can contribute to Leaky Gut Syndrome by disrupting the balance of microorganisms in the gut.

5. **Environmental Toxins:** Exposure to environmental toxins, such as pesticides and pollutants, can have a negative impact on gut health and increase the risk of a leaky gut.

6. **Genetics:** Some individuals may be genetically predisposed to a weaker gut barrier, making them more susceptible to Leaky Gut Syndrome.

7. **Chronic Illness:** Certain chronic conditions, such as Crohn's disease and celiac disease, are associated with increased intestinal permeability.

Recognizing Symptoms of Leaky Gut Syndrome

Leaky Gut Syndrome is often called a "silent" condition because its symptoms can vary widely and mimic those of other health issues. Recognizing these symptoms is crucial for early detection and intervention. Common symptoms include:

- **Digestive Issues:** These may include gas, bloating, diarrhea, and irritable bowel syndrome (IBS)-like symptoms.
- **Food Sensitivities:** People with Leaky Gut Syndrome often develop sensitivities or intolerances to certain foods, particularly gluten and dairy.
- **Skin Problems:** Skin conditions like acne, eczema,

and psoriasis can be exacerbated by a leaky gut.

- **Autoimmune Conditions:** There's growing evidence that Leaky Gut Syndrome may play a role in the development or exacerbation of autoimmune diseases like rheumatoid arthritis and lupus.

- **Mood Disorders:** Some individuals with a leaky gut experience mood swings, anxiety, and even depression. The gut-brain connection is a fascinating area of research, and an imbalanced gut can affect your mental well-being.

- **Allergies and Asthma:** A compromised gut barrier may contribute to an increase in allergies and asthma symptoms.

- **Chronic Fatigue:** Fatigue and low energy levels are common complaints among those with Leaky Gut Syndrome.

- **Nutritional Deficiencies:** Malabsorption due to a damaged gut lining can lead to nutrient deficiencies.

- **Joint Pain:** Conditions like joint pain and arthritis can be linked to inflammation in the gut.

The Importance of Addressing Leaky Gut

You might be wondering why it's so crucial to address Leaky Gut Syndrome. The answer lies in the far-reaching consequences it can have on your health.

First and foremost, a leaky gut can contribute to chronic inflammation throughout the body. Chronic inflammation is now recognized as a driving force behind many chronic diseases, including heart disease, diabetes, and cancer. So, by addressing the root cause of this inflammation – a leaky gut – you're taking a significant step towards preventing or managing these conditions.

Additionally, the gut is often referred to as the "second brain" because of the strong connection between the gut and the brain. When your gut is out of balance, it can affect your mood and mental health. Treating Leaky Gut Syndrome can lead to improvements in anxiety, depression, and overall emotional well-being.

Furthermore, a healthy gut is essential for a robust immune system. The gut houses a significant portion of your immune cells, and a leaky gut can lead to immune dysfunction. By repairing your gut, you're bolstering your body's natural defenses against infections and illnesses.

In summary, Leaky Gut Syndrome is not a condition to be taken lightly. It has far-reaching effects on your health and well-being, impacting everything from digestion and allergies to mental health and chronic disease risk.

Understanding the causes and symptoms of Leaky Gut Syndrome is the first step toward healing your gut and improving your overall health.

In the following chapters, we'll delve into practical steps you can take to address Leaky Gut Syndrome, including dietary changes, supplements, and lifestyle modifications. By the end of this book, you'll have the knowledge and tools to embark on a journey to heal your gut and enhance your quality of life.

CHAPTER 2

The Gut-Health Connection

In this chapter, we'll embark on a fascinating exploration of the intricate relationship between your gut and your overall health. Understanding this connection is essential because it lays the foundation for comprehending why a leaky gut can have such a profound impact on your well-being.

The Gut Microbiome: Your Gut's Ecosystem

At the heart of the gut-health connection is a bustling, microscopic world known as the gut microbiome. Picture this: your gastrointestinal tract, from your mouth to your colon, is home to trillions of microorganisms, including bacteria, viruses, fungi, and more. Collectively, these microorganisms form what scientists often refer to as the gut microbiome.

This gut ecosystem is not just a random collection of microbes; it's a highly organized and complex community. Each microbe plays a unique role in maintaining your health. Some are beneficial, while others can be harmful if they overpopulate or become imbalanced.

The Gut Microbiome and Your Immune System

One of the most remarkable aspects of the gut microbiome is its profound influence on your immune system. It's no exaggeration to say that a significant portion of your immune cells resides in your gut. This makes sense when you consider that your gut is one of the primary entry points for potential invaders like bacteria and viruses.

Your gut microbiome acts as a barrier, protecting your body from harmful pathogens. Beneficial bacteria, also known as probiotics, help maintain this barrier by crowding out potential troublemakers and producing compounds that inhibit their growth.

However, when the balance of beneficial and harmful bacteria in your gut is disrupted – a condition known as dysbiosis – your gut's protective barrier can weaken. This can lead to increased susceptibility to infections and contribute to inflammatory conditions.

The Gut-Brain Axis: Your Second Brain

Beyond its role in immunity, your gut also communicates closely with your brain, forming a bidirectional connection known as the gut-brain axis. This connection is a two-way street, with signals constantly traveling back and forth between your gut and your brain.

For example, have you ever experienced "butterflies in your stomach" before a big event? That's your gut-brain axis at work.

Emotions like stress and anxiety can influence the function of your gut, leading to those familiar feelings of unease.

Conversely, the health of your gut can influence your mental well-being. Research has shown that imbalances in the gut microbiome can be linked to mood disorders like anxiety and depression. The gut produces neurotransmitters, such as serotonin (often referred to as the "feel-good" neurotransmitter), that can influence your mood and emotional state.

The Gut-Health Connection and Chronic Inflammation

Perhaps one of the most significant revelations in recent years is how the gut-health connection ties into chronic inflammation – a key player in many chronic diseases.

When the gut microbiome becomes imbalanced or when the gut lining is compromised (as in Leaky Gut Syndrome), harmful substances can pass through the intestinal barrier and enter your bloodstream. Your immune system detects these intruders and mounts an inflammatory response to neutralize them.

While this inflammatory response is a natural defense mechanism, chronic inflammation – when it persists over long periods – is detrimental to your health. It's like a low-grade fire that can smolder in your body, damaging tissues and organs. Chronic inflammation is now recognized as a common thread in conditions ranging from heart disease and diabetes to cancer and neurodegenerative diseases like Alzheimer's.

So, how does a leaky gut contribute to chronic

inflammation? The answer lies in a concept called "endotoxemia." When harmful substances, such as bacterial fragments or toxins, leak into your bloodstream through a compromised gut barrier, they can trigger an immune response and elevate inflammation levels. This ongoing inflammation can fuel the development and progression of chronic diseases.

The Gut-Health Connection and Nutrient Absorption

Your gut is not only responsible for keeping harmful substances out but also for absorbing the essential nutrients your body needs to function optimally. A healthy gut lining is lined with tiny hair-like structures called villi and microvilli that increase the surface area for nutrient absorption.

However, when your gut lining is damaged – as it is in Leaky Gut Syndrome – this critical function can be impaired. Malabsorption of nutrients, even when you're eating a balanced diet, can lead to nutrient deficiencies. These deficiencies can have wide-ranging effects on your health, from weakened bones (due to calcium and vitamin D deficiencies) to compromised immune function (due to insufficient vitamins and minerals).

The Gut-Health Connection and Food Sensitivities

Another crucial aspect of the gut-health connection is its role in the development of food sensitivities and intolerances. When your gut is compromised, it becomes more permeable, allowing larger food particles to enter your bloodstream. Your immune system may identify these particles as threats and mount an immune response against them.

Over time, this immune response can lead to the development of food sensitivities, where your body reacts adversely to specific foods. Gluten and dairy are common culprits, but virtually any food can become a trigger. These sensitivities can cause digestive discomfort, skin issues, headaches, and other symptoms.

In Conclusion: The Gut-Health Connection is Central to Your Well-Being

The gut-health connection is a remarkably intricate and vital aspect of your overall health. Your gut microbiome influences your immune system, communicates with your brain, plays a role in chronic inflammation, affects nutrient absorption, and can lead to food sensitivities.

Understanding this connection is the key to grasping why a leaky gut can have such profound and widespread effects on your well-being. In the following chapters, we'll delve into practical steps you can take to restore and maintain a healthy gut, including dietary choices, nutritional supplements, and lifestyle modifications. Armed with this knowledge, you'll be better equipped to embark on your journey towards healing your gut and enhancing your overall health.

CHAPTER 3

Identifying Problematic Foods

In Chapter 3, we delve into a critical aspect of managing Leaky Gut Syndrome: identifying and understanding problematic foods. Leaky Gut Syndrome is closely tied to the foods you consume, and recognizing which foods may be exacerbating your condition is a crucial step toward healing.

The Role of Diet in Leaky Gut Syndrome

Before we dive into specifics, it's essential to understand the intimate connection between your diet and the health of your gut lining. Your gastrointestinal tract is the frontline of interaction between your body and the outside world, particularly the food you eat. It's responsible for processing and absorbing nutrients while keeping harmful substances out.

However, in Leaky Gut Syndrome, this protective barrier is compromised. Gaps or "leaks" form in the gut lining, allowing undigested food particles, toxins, and bacteria to slip through into your bloodstream. This can lead to immune reactions and inflammation, further weakening the gut lining and perpetuating the cycle.

Common Trigger Foods for Leaky Gut

Not all foods are created equal when it comes to their impact on a leaky gut. Some foods are more likely to contribute to inflammation and exacerbate your symptoms. While individual sensitivities can vary, certain categories of foods are commonly associated with Leaky Gut Syndrome:

1. **Gluten:** Gluten is a protein found in wheat, barley, rye, and many processed foods. It's a well-known trigger for gut inflammation and is often problematic for individuals with Leaky Gut Syndrome.

2. **Dairy:** Lactose, a sugar found in dairy products, and casein, a protein in milk, can be challenging for those with compromised gut health.

3. **Processed Foods:** Highly processed foods, rich in sugar, unhealthy fats, and artificial additives, can

contribute to gut inflammation.

4. **Sugars and Artificial Sweeteners:** Excessive sugar intake and artificial sweeteners like aspartame and sucralose can disrupt the balance of gut bacteria and promote inflammation.

5. **Alcohol:** Excessive alcohol consumption can damage the gut lining and contribute to inflammation.

6. **Caffeine:** While moderate caffeine intake may be fine for some, excessive consumption can irritate the gut lining.

7. **Nightshades:** Some individuals with Leaky Gut Syndrome are sensitive to nightshade vegetables like tomatoes, peppers, and eggplants.

8. **Highly Allergenic Foods:** Shellfish, peanuts, and tree nuts can be problematic for those with food allergies or sensitivities.

9. **Processed Vegetable Oils:** Oils like soybean, corn, and canola oil, which are commonly used in processed foods, are high in pro-inflammatory omega-6 fatty acids.

Recognizing Food Sensitivities

Identifying which specific foods trigger your symptoms can be a bit of detective work, as reactions can vary from person to person. Here are some common ways to recognize food sensitivities:

1. **Food Diary:** Keeping a detailed food diary can help you track what you eat and any symptoms that arise. Look for patterns over time to identify potential triggers.

2. **Elimination Diet:** An elimination diet involves removing common trigger

foods from your diet for a specified period, then reintroducing them one by one while monitoring for symptoms. This can help pinpoint problematic foods.

3. **Lab Testing:** Some lab tests, like food sensitivity tests or IgG antibody tests, can provide insights into specific foods that might be causing issues. However, these tests are not always definitive and should be interpreted alongside clinical symptoms.

4. **Working with a Healthcare Professional:**

A healthcare professional, such as a registered dietitian or functional medicine practitioner, can provide guidance and support in identifying food sensitivities.

The Role of Gluten and Dairy

Gluten and dairy deserve special attention due to their frequent association with Leaky Gut Syndrome.

Gluten: Gluten is a protein found in wheat, barley, rye, and their derivatives. It's a well-documented trigger for inflammation and gut-related conditions. In individuals with Leaky Gut Syndrome, gluten can be particularly problematic.

One reason for this is a protein called zonulin, which regulates the tight junctions between the cells of the intestinal lining. Gluten has been shown to increase the release of zonulin, potentially leading to increased intestinal permeability. This is why many individuals with Leaky Gut Syndrome find relief by adopting a gluten-free diet.

Dairy: Dairy products contain two main components that can be problematic for some: lactose and casein. Lactose intolerance, the inability to digest lactose, is relatively common. In Leaky Gut Syndrome, the damaged gut lining may struggle to produce sufficient lactase, the enzyme needed to digest lactose.

Casein, on the other hand, is a protein in milk that can cross-react with gluten antibodies. This means that if you're sensitive to gluten, you might also react to casein. Some individuals with Leaky Gut Syndrome find relief by eliminating dairy from their diet.

Navigating Your Leaky Gut Diet

Crafting a diet that supports your gut healing is a personalized journey. Once you've identified trigger foods, the next step is to build a diet that nourishes your body and promotes gut health. This typically involves:

1. **Incorporating Gut-Friendly Foods:** Emphasize foods that are easy on the gut, such as cooked vegetables, lean proteins, and sources of healthy fats like avocados and olive oil.

2. **Including Fermented Foods:** Fermented foods

like yogurt (if tolerated), kefir, sauerkraut, and kimchi contain beneficial probiotics that can support a healthy gut microbiome.

3. **Prioritizing Fiber:** Fiber-rich foods, including fruits, vegetables, and whole grains (if tolerated), can support digestive regularity and feed beneficial gut bacteria.

4. **Hydrating Adequately:** Staying hydrated is crucial for maintaining gut health and ensuring that digestive processes run smoothly.

5. **Limiting Processed Foods:** Minimize processed

and sugary foods that can promote inflammation and disrupt the balance of gut bacteria.

6. **Managing Portion Sizes:** Overeating can place additional stress on your digestive system. Be mindful of portion sizes to support your gut's recovery.

7. **Staying Consistent:** Consistency in your diet is key. Gradual changes are often more sustainable and allow your gut to adapt.

In Conclusion: Identifying and Managing Problematic Foods

In Chapter 3, we've explored the significance of recognizing problematic foods in the context of Leaky Gut Syndrome. Your diet plays a pivotal role in the health of your gut lining, and certain foods can exacerbate inflammation and symptoms.

By identifying trigger foods through methods like food diaries, elimination diets, lab testing, or professional guidance, you can take control of your diet and begin the process of healing your gut.

Tailoring your diet to support gut health with the inclusion of gut-friendly foods, probiotics, fiber, and adequate hydration is a crucial step in your journey toward better health and relief from Leaky Gut Syndrome.

CHAPTER 4

The Leaky Gut Diet Plan

In Chapter 4, we embark on a practical journey toward healing your gut through a comprehensive Leaky Gut Diet Plan. This plan focuses on foods to include for gut healing, foods to avoid, meal planning, and even provides you with some delicious recipes to get started.

Foods to Include for Healing

When you're dealing with Leaky Gut Syndrome, it's crucial to choose foods that support the repair and maintenance of your gut lining. Here are some key elements to include in your Leaky Gut Diet:

1. **Non-Starchy Vegetables:** Vegetables like leafy greens, broccoli, cauliflower, and carrots are rich in fiber, vitamins, and minerals that promote gut health.

2. **Lean Proteins:** Incorporate sources of lean protein, such as chicken, turkey, fish, and tofu. Protein is essential for tissue repair and overall health.

3. **Bone Broth:** Bone broth is packed with nutrients like collagen and amino acids that can help repair the gut lining.

4. **Fermented Foods:** Yogurt (if tolerated), kefir, sauerkraut, kimchi, and kombucha contain beneficial probiotics that support a healthy gut microbiome.

5. **Healthy Fats:** Include sources of healthy fats like avocados, olive oil, and fatty fish (e.g., salmon and mackerel). These fats provide essential nutrients for gut health.

6. **Fiber-Rich Foods:**
Consume foods high in
soluble fiber, such as oats,
chia seeds, and flaxseeds.
Soluble fiber supports
digestive regularity and
feeds beneficial gut bacteria.

7. **Herbs and Spices:**
Incorporate herbs and spices
like turmeric, ginger, and
oregano, which have anti-
inflammatory and digestive
properties.

8. **Low-Sugar Fruits:** Opt for
fruits that are lower in sugar,
such as berries, apples, and
pears. These can provide

essential nutrients without spiking blood sugar.

9. **Nuts and Seeds:** Almonds, walnuts, and seeds like pumpkin and sunflower seeds can be part of a gut-friendly diet when consumed in moderation.

10. **Coconut Products:** Coconut oil, coconut milk, and coconut flour are often well-tolerated and can be used in cooking and baking.

Foods to Avoid

Equally important to the foods you include in your Leaky Gut Diet are those you should avoid or limit.

These items can exacerbate inflammation and worsen gut symptoms:

1. **Gluten-Containing Foods:** Eliminate or significantly reduce foods with gluten, including wheat, barley, and rye.

2. **Dairy Products:** If you're sensitive to dairy, avoid or limit milk, cheese, and yogurt. Consider dairy-free alternatives like almond or coconut milk.

3. **Processed Foods:** Stay away from highly processed foods, which often contain

unhealthy fats, additives, and preservatives.

4. **Added Sugars:** Minimize your consumption of added sugars, including sugary drinks, candies, and desserts.

5. **Alcohol:** If possible, avoid alcohol or limit your intake. Alcohol can irritate the gut lining and disrupt the gut microbiome.

6. **Caffeine:** Cut back on caffeine if you find that it irritates your gut. Opt for herbal teas or decaffeinated coffee instead.

7. **Artificial Sweeteners:** Steer clear of artificial sweeteners like aspartame and sucralose, which can negatively impact gut health.

8. **Processed Vegetable Oils:** Avoid oils like soybean, corn, and canola oil, which are high in pro-inflammatory omega-6 fatty acids.

9. **Highly Spiced Foods:** For some individuals, highly spiced foods can irritate the gut. Pay attention to how your body reacts to spices.

10. **Nightshade Vegetables:** If you suspect

nightshades are problematic for you, consider eliminating them temporarily to see if your symptoms improve.

Meal Planning for Gut Health

Creating balanced, gut-friendly meals is an essential part of the Leaky Gut Diet Plan. Here's how to structure your meals for maximum benefit:

Breakfast:

- Start your day with a gut-healing smoothie made with leafy greens, frozen berries, a scoop of collagen powder, and almond milk.

- Alternatively, enjoy a bowl of overnight oats topped with chia seeds, chopped nuts, and a drizzle of honey (if tolerated).

Lunch:

- Opt for a salad with plenty of non-starchy vegetables, grilled chicken or tofu, and a homemade vinaigrette dressing made with olive oil and herbs.
- Consider a bowl of vegetable soup with a side of fermented kimchi or sauerkraut.

Snacks:

- Choose gut-friendly snacks like a small handful of mixed nuts, carrot sticks with hummus, or a serving of Greek yogurt (if tolerated).

Dinner:

- Prepare a baked salmon fillet with a side of steamed broccoli and quinoa.
- For a vegetarian option, make a stir-fry with tofu, bell peppers, and bok choy in a ginger-turmeric sauce served over brown rice.

Dessert (in moderation):

- Satisfy your sweet tooth with a small serving of fresh berries drizzled with a touch of honey or a square of dark chocolate.

Hydration:

- Stay well-hydrated throughout the day by drinking water, herbal teas, or infused water with cucumber and mint.

Recipes for Gut Healing

To kickstart your Leaky Gut Diet Plan, here are a couple of gut-friendly recipes:

1. **Gut-Healing Chicken and Vegetable Soup** Ingredients:

- 2 boneless, skinless chicken breasts
- 6 cups chicken broth (homemade or low-sodium)
- 2 carrots, peeled and chopped
- 2 celery stalks, chopped
- 1 onion, diced
- 2 cloves garlic, minced
- 1 teaspoon turmeric
- 1 teaspoon ginger
- Salt and pepper to taste
- Fresh parsley, chopped (for garnish)

Instructions:

1. In a large pot, sauté the onion, garlic, carrots, and celery in a bit of olive oil until softened.

2. Add the chicken breasts, chicken broth, turmeric, ginger, salt, and pepper.

3. Bring to a boil, then reduce heat, cover, and simmer for about 20-25 minutes, or until the chicken is cooked through.

4. Remove the chicken, shred it with two forks, and return it to the pot.

5. Serve hot, garnished with fresh parsley.

2. Berry and Chia Seed Parfait Ingredients:

- 1 cup mixed berries (strawberries, blueberries, raspberries)
- 2 tablespoons chia seeds
- 1 cup Greek yogurt (if tolerated) or dairy-free yogurt
- 1 tablespoon honey (optional)
- 1/4 cup chopped nuts (almonds or walnuts)

Instructions:

1. In a bowl, mix the chia seeds and yogurt. If using, add honey for sweetness.

2. Layer the chia-yogurt mixture with the mixed berries in a glass or jar.

3. Top with chopped nuts for crunch and additional nutrients.

4. Refrigerate for at least 2 hours or overnight before enjoying.

In Conclusion: A Practical Leaky Gut Diet Plan

Chapter 4 has provided you with a practical Leaky Gut Diet Plan to help you navigate the journey to healing your gut. By including gut-friendly foods, avoiding problematic ones, and planning balanced meals, you can take significant steps toward improving your gut health and overall well-being.

Remember that this plan is a starting point, and it's essential to listen to your body's signals. Pay attention to how specific foods affect you and make adjustments accordingly. In the following chapters, we'll explore additional strategies, including nutritional supplements and lifestyle modifications, to further support your gut healing journey. With dedication and a well-planned diet, you're well on your way to a healthier gut and a better quality of life.

CHAPTER 5

Nutritional Supplements for Gut Health

In this chapter, we will explore the role of nutritional supplements in supporting gut health, especially when dealing with Leaky Gut Syndrome. While a well-balanced diet is fundamental to healing your gut, certain supplements can provide targeted support to expedite the healing process and maintain long-term gut health.

1. Probiotics

Probiotics are beneficial bacteria that play a crucial role in maintaining a healthy gut microbiome. They can help restore balance to your gut by increasing the population of friendly bacteria. These supplements come in various strains and forms, including capsules, powders, and fermented foods.

- **Lactobacillus acidophilus:** This strain is known for its ability to support digestive health and may help alleviate symptoms like gas and bloating.

- **Bifidobacterium bifidum:** It can help regulate bowel movements and reduce inflammation in the gut.

- **Saccharomyces boulardii:** This yeast-based probiotic can be beneficial in treating diarrhea and other digestive issues.

When selecting a probiotic supplement, it's important to choose one with strains that are suited to your specific needs. Consulting a healthcare professional can help you determine the most appropriate probiotic for your condition.

2. Prebiotics

Prebiotics are non-digestible fibers that serve as food for beneficial gut bacteria. They can help create an environment conducive to the growth and activity of probiotics. Some common prebiotic supplements include:

- **Inulin:** A soluble fiber found in many plants, including chicory root and artichokes, inulin is commonly used as a prebiotic supplement.

- **Fructo-oligosaccharides (FOS):** These short-chain carbohydrates are naturally present in certain foods and can be taken as supplements to support gut health.

By providing nourishment for your beneficial gut bacteria, prebiotics can enhance the effectiveness of probiotics and contribute to a healthier gut microbiome.

3. Digestive Enzymes

Digestive enzymes are essential for breaking down food into its component nutrients, making them more easily absorbed by your body. In cases of Leaky Gut Syndrome, where digestion may be compromised, digestive enzyme supplements can be helpful. Common enzymes include:

- **Lipase:** Breaks down fats into fatty acids and glycerol.

- **Amylase:** Helps digest carbohydrates into simple sugars.

- **Protease:** Aids in protein digestion, breaking them down into amino acids.

- **Cellulase:** Breaks down cellulose, a plant fiber.

These supplements can assist your body in the digestion and

absorption of nutrients, reducing the workload on your gut.

4. L-Glutamine

L-glutamine is an amino acid known for its role in maintaining the integrity of the gut lining. It serves as a primary energy source for the cells that make up the intestinal barrier. When taken as a supplement, L-glutamine can help repair and strengthen the gut lining, potentially reducing permeability. It may also help alleviate symptoms associated with Leaky Gut Syndrome, such as diarrhea and abdominal pain.

5. Collagen

Collagen is a structural protein that plays a vital role in the health of your gut lining, as well as your skin, hair, and joints. Collagen supplements, typically derived from animal sources, can provide the amino acids necessary for tissue repair and regeneration. Collagen peptides are a popular form of this supplement and are easily absorbed by the body.

By supporting the healing and maintenance of the gut lining, collagen supplements can be a valuable addition to your gut health regimen.

6. Zinc

Zinc is a mineral that plays a critical role in maintaining the integrity of the gut lining. It supports the repair of damaged tissues and contributes to the overall health of the mucosal lining in the gastrointestinal tract. Zinc supplements may be beneficial for individuals with Leaky Gut Syndrome, especially if they are deficient in this essential nutrient.

7. Fish Oil (Omega-3 Fatty Acids)

Omega-3 fatty acids, commonly found in fish oil supplements, have anti-inflammatory properties. They can help reduce inflammation in the gut, which is often a significant factor in Leaky Gut Syndrome and other digestive disorders. Omega-3 supplements may also support the overall health of the gut lining.

8. Quercetin

Quercetin is a flavonoid found in certain fruits and vegetables. It has antioxidant and anti-inflammatory properties and may help stabilize mast cells in the gut, which can reduce symptoms of gut inflammation and irritation.

9. Marshmallow Root

Marshmallow root is an herbal supplement known for its mucilaginous properties. It can help soothe and coat the lining of the digestive tract, potentially reducing irritation and inflammation. It's often used to alleviate symptoms of digestive discomfort.

10. Aloe Vera

Aloe vera supplements, derived from the inner gel of the aloe plant, can have soothing effects on the digestive tract. Aloe vera contains compounds that may help reduce inflammation and support gut healing.

Consultation with a Healthcare Professional

Before adding any nutritional supplements to your regimen, it's essential to consult with a healthcare professional, such as a doctor or registered dietitian. They can help you determine which supplements are appropriate for your specific condition, dosage guidelines, and potential interactions with medications.

In Conclusion: Supplements for Gut Health

Chapter 5 has explored various nutritional supplements that can play a supportive role in healing and maintaining gut health, particularly when dealing with Leaky Gut Syndrome. These supplements can aid in restoring the gut microbiome, repairing the gut lining, and reducing inflammation.

However, supplements should not be viewed as a standalone solution but as part of a comprehensive approach that includes dietary changes and lifestyle modifications. The synergy between a gut-friendly diet, proper supplementation, and lifestyle adjustments can significantly enhance your efforts to heal your gut and promote long-term well-being.

In the following chapters, we will delve into lifestyle changes, stress management, exercise, and other factors that contribute to gut health, creating a holistic approach to improving your overall digestive wellness.

CHAPTER 6

Lifestyle Modifications for Gut Health

In this chapter, we delve into the critical role of lifestyle modifications in supporting and maintaining gut health, especially when dealing with Leaky Gut Syndrome. While dietary choices and nutritional supplements are essential components of gut health, lifestyle factors can profoundly influence the state of your gut and its ability to heal.

1. Stress Management

Stress is a well-known disruptor of gut health. The gut-brain connection, often referred to as the gut-brain axis, highlights the intricate relationship between your emotional well-being and digestive health. Chronic stress can lead to a range of gastrointestinal issues, including increased permeability of the gut lining.

Mindfulness and Relaxation Techniques: Practices like mindfulness meditation, deep breathing exercises, and progressive muscle relaxation can help reduce stress levels and promote a more balanced gut environment. Engaging in these techniques regularly can be a valuable addition to your daily routine.

Regular Exercise: Physical activity has been shown to reduce stress and improve mood, both of which can benefit gut health. Aim for regular, moderate exercise, such as brisk walking, yoga, or swimming, to help manage stress levels.

Adequate Sleep: Sleep is essential for overall health, including gut health. Aim for 7-9 hours of quality sleep per night to support your body's repair and maintenance processes, including gut healing.

2. Adequate Hydration

Proper hydration is crucial for digestive wellness. Water helps transport nutrients, supports the elimination of waste products, and maintains the mucosal lining of the gastrointestinal tract. Insufficient hydration can lead to constipation and hinder the body's natural detoxification processes.

Water Intake: Ensure you're drinking enough water throughout the day. General guidelines recommend around 8 cups (64 ounces) of water daily, but individual needs may vary based on factors like climate and physical activity.

Herbal Teas: Herbal teas like ginger, peppermint, and chamomile can be soothing to the digestive system and contribute to overall hydration.

3. Adequate Fiber Intake

Fiber is a cornerstone of gut health, as it supports regular bowel movements and provides nourishment for beneficial gut bacteria. Insufficient fiber intake can lead to constipation and an imbalanced gut microbiome.

Fiber-Rich Foods: Incorporate a variety of fiber-rich foods into your diet, including fruits, vegetables, whole grains (if tolerated), legumes, and nuts. These foods provide both soluble and insoluble fiber, benefiting overall digestive health.

Gradual Increase: If you're not used to a high-fiber diet, introduce fiber gradually to allow your gut to adapt. Sudden increases in fiber intake can lead to digestive discomfort.

4. Limit Antibiotic Use

Antibiotics can be lifesaving medications, but they can also disrupt the balance of beneficial gut bacteria. Overuse or unnecessary use of antibiotics can have a long-lasting impact on gut health. If you're prescribed antibiotics, discuss with your healthcare provider the possibility of taking probiotics alongside them to help mitigate the disruption.

5. Avoid Environmental Toxins

Exposure to environmental toxins, such as pesticides and pollutants, can negatively impact gut health. These toxins can disrupt the balance of gut bacteria and contribute to inflammation in the gastrointestinal tract.

Organic Foods: Whenever possible, choose organic foods to reduce your exposure to pesticides and herbicides commonly found on conventionally grown produce.

Filtered Water: Use a water filter to reduce the presence of contaminants in your drinking water.

Limit Toxin Exposure: Be mindful of environmental toxins in your everyday life, such as household cleaning products and personal care items. Opt for natural, eco-friendly alternatives when possible.

6. Limit Alcohol and Caffeine

Excessive alcohol and caffeine consumption can irritate the gut lining and disrupt gut health. While moderate consumption of these substances may be acceptable for some, it's essential to pay attention to how your body reacts.

Moderation: If you choose to consume alcohol and caffeine, do so in moderation and be mindful of any adverse effects on your gut and overall well-being.

7. Practice Food Hygiene

Practicing proper food hygiene can reduce the risk of foodborne illnesses that can damage the gut and disrupt gut flora. Follow these guidelines:

Food Storage: Store food at the appropriate temperatures to prevent bacterial growth.

Food Handling: Wash your hands and food preparation

surfaces regularly to avoid contamination.

Proper Cooking: Cook foods thoroughly to kill harmful bacteria.

8. Stay Informed and Seek Professional Guidance

Staying informed about the latest research and developments in gut health can empower you to make informed choices. However, it's crucial to remember that individual responses to lifestyle modifications can vary significantly. Seek professional guidance from a healthcare provider, such as a gastroenterologist or registered dietitian, to create a tailored plan that suits your unique needs.

In Conclusion: A Holistic Approach to Gut Health

Chapter 6 has explored the critical role of lifestyle modifications in supporting and maintaining gut health. These modifications encompass stress management, hydration, fiber intake, antibiotic use, toxin exposure, alcohol and caffeine consumption, food hygiene, and staying informed.

While dietary choices and nutritional supplements are essential components of gut health, lifestyle factors are equally influential. The synergy between a gut-friendly diet, proper supplementation, and lifestyle adjustments creates a holistic approach to improving your overall digestive wellness and managing conditions like Leaky Gut Syndrome.

In the following chapters, we will delve into additional aspects of gut health, including the impact of chronic inflammation, immune system support, and practical tips for long-term gut maintenance. Armed with a comprehensive understanding of these factors, you'll be better equipped to nurture a healthy gut and enhance your overall quality of life.

CHAPTER 7

Long-Term Gut Maintenance and a Healthier You

In this final chapter, we explore the key principles of long-term gut maintenance and how they contribute to overall well-being. By adopting these practices, you can sustain the progress you've made in healing your gut and continue on a path to a healthier, happier you.

1. Maintain a Gut-Friendly Diet

A gut-friendly diet is not just a short-term solution; it's a way of eating that can support your gut health for the long term. Continue to emphasize foods that promote a healthy gut microbiome, such as:

- **Fiber-rich Foods:** Fruits, vegetables, whole grains, legumes, and nuts should be staples in your diet. These provide essential nutrients and nourish beneficial gut bacteria.

- **Lean Proteins:** Include sources of lean protein like poultry, fish, tofu, and beans. Protein is vital for tissue repair and overall health.

- **Healthy Fats:** Incorporate healthy fats from sources like avocados, olive oil, and fatty fish. These fats provide essential nutrients for gut health.

- **Fermented Foods:** Continue to enjoy fermented foods like yogurt (if tolerated), kefir, sauerkraut, kimchi, and kombucha to support a diverse gut microbiome.

- **Low-Sugar Fruits:** Choose fruits that are lower in sugar, such as berries, apples, and pears, for essential nutrients without spiking blood sugar.

- **Herbs and Spices:** Use herbs and spices like turmeric, ginger, and oregano, which have anti-inflammatory and digestive properties.

2. Stay Hydrated

Proper hydration is vital for digestive wellness and overall health. Continue to drink an adequate amount of water daily. Herbal teas can also contribute to your hydration needs while offering additional digestive benefits.

3. Manage Stress

Chronic stress can have a significant impact on gut health, so it's essential to incorporate stress management techniques into your daily life for the long term:

- **Mindfulness and Relaxation:** Continue mindfulness meditation, deep breathing exercises, or progressive muscle relaxation to reduce stress levels.
- **Regular Exercise:** Maintain a routine of regular, moderate exercise to

help manage stress and improve mood.

- **Adequate Sleep:** Prioritize quality sleep, aiming for 7-9 hours per night, to support overall health and well-being.

4. Incorporate Probiotics and Prebiotics

Probiotics and prebiotics are valuable for ongoing gut health. Consider integrating probiotic-rich foods into your diet and continue taking probiotic supplements if recommended by your healthcare provider.

5. Limit Antibiotics

Whenever possible, avoid unnecessary or excessive use of antibiotics. If you require antibiotics for a medical condition, discuss with your healthcare provider the possibility of taking probiotics alongside them to help maintain a balanced gut microbiome.

6. Be Mindful of Toxin Exposure

Maintain awareness of environmental toxins in your surroundings and continue to make choices that reduce your exposure, such as using organic foods and filtered water. Be conscious of toxins in household cleaning products and personal care items and opt for natural alternatives.

7. Moderation with Alcohol and Caffeine

If you choose to consume alcohol and caffeine, do so in moderation and be aware of their effects on your gut and overall well-being.

8. Prioritize Food Hygiene

Continue to practice proper food hygiene, including safe food storage, regular hand washing, and thorough cooking to prevent foodborne illnesses.

9. Seek Professional Guidance and Monitoring

Regular check-ins with a healthcare provider, such as a gastroenterologist or registered dietitian, can be valuable for monitoring your gut health and making adjustments to your plan as needed. They can provide guidance on any necessary dietary modifications, supplementation, and lifestyle changes.

10. Listen to Your Body

One of the most important aspects of long-term gut maintenance is listening to your body's signals. Pay attention to how specific foods affect you, monitor any changes in your digestive health, and make adjustments accordingly. Your body is an excellent guide for what works best for you.

11. Be Patient and Consistent

Healing and maintaining gut health is often a journey that requires patience and consistency. While you may experience improvements early on, it's important to continue your efforts over the long term to sustain the benefits.

12. Embrace a Holistic Approach to Health

Remember that gut health is interconnected with overall health. A holistic approach to wellness includes not only dietary choices but also stress management, adequate sleep, regular exercise, and emotional well-being. By nurturing your body as a whole, you support the health of your gut.

CONCLUSION

A Healthier You through Long-Term Gut Maintenance

Chapter 7 has explored the principles of long-term gut maintenance and how they contribute to overall well-being. By maintaining a gut-friendly diet, staying hydrated, managing stress, incorporating probiotics and prebiotics, and being mindful of toxins and other lifestyle factors, you can sustain the progress you've made in healing your gut.

Remember that gut health is an ongoing journey, and your body is unique. What works for one person may not work for another, so it's essential to tailor your approach based on your individual needs and responses.

With dedication and a holistic approach to health, you can continue to nurture a healthy gut, reduce the risk of digestive issues, and enjoy a higher quality of life. Gut health is at the core of your overall well-being, and by prioritizing it, you're investing in your long-term health and happiness.

In conclusion, the journey to understanding and improving

your gut health, especially when dealing with conditions like Leaky Gut Syndrome, is a multifaceted process that requires dedication, patience, and a holistic approach. Here's a summary of the key takeaways from our exploration of the seven chapters:

Chapter 1: Introduction to Leaky Gut Syndrome

- Leaky Gut Syndrome is a condition characterized by increased intestinal permeability.
- It can lead to a range of health issues, from digestive

problems to systemic inflammation.

- Understanding the basics of your gut's structure and function is crucial for managing this condition.

Chapter 2: The Gut-Body Connection

- The gut plays a central role in overall health, influencing not only digestion but also the immune system, mood, and more.

- An imbalance in the gut microbiome can contribute to health problems beyond digestive issues.

- The gut-brain axis highlights the connection between gut health and emotional well-being.

Chapter 3: Identifying Problematic Foods

- Recognizing problematic foods is essential for managing Leaky Gut Syndrome.
- Common trigger foods include gluten, dairy, processed foods, sugars, and more.
- Identifying food sensitivities through methods like food

diaries and elimination diets is crucial.

Chapter 4: The Leaky Gut Diet Plan

- The Leaky Gut Diet Plan focuses on including gut-friendly foods and avoiding trigger foods.
- Meal planning, recipes, and balanced nutrition are key components of this plan.
- Hydration, portion control, and consistency in your diet are essential for success.

Chapter 5: Nutritional Supplements for Gut Health

- Nutritional supplements like probiotics, prebiotics, and digestive enzymes can support gut healing.

- Specific supplements like L-glutamine, collagen, and fish oil target gut lining repair and inflammation reduction.

- Consulting a healthcare professional is essential before adding supplements to your regimen.

Chapter 6: Lifestyle Modifications for Gut Health

- Lifestyle factors such as stress management,

hydration, and exercise are integral to gut health.

- Adequate sleep, toxin avoidance, and mindful alcohol and caffeine consumption contribute to a healthy gut.
- Proper food hygiene and staying informed are crucial for ongoing gut wellness.

Chapter 7: Long-Term Gut Maintenance and a Healthier You

- Maintaining a gut-friendly diet, staying hydrated, and managing stress are ongoing practices for gut health.

- Probiotics, prebiotics, and avoiding excessive antibiotic use are essential for a balanced gut microbiome.

- Regular check-ins with healthcare professionals, listening to your body, and embracing a holistic approach are key for long-term gut maintenance.

Incorporating these principles into your daily life can lead to a healthier gut and, consequently, a healthier you. Gut health is intimately linked to overall well-being, and by prioritizing it, you're investing in your long-term health, happiness, and quality of life.

Remember that everyone's journey to optimal gut health is unique, and it may take time to find the right combination of dietary choices, supplements, and lifestyle adjustments that work best for you. Be patient, stay consistent, and seek professional guidance as needed. Your gut health is a vital foundation for a vibrant and fulfilling life.